YOUR KNOWLEDGE HAS VALUE

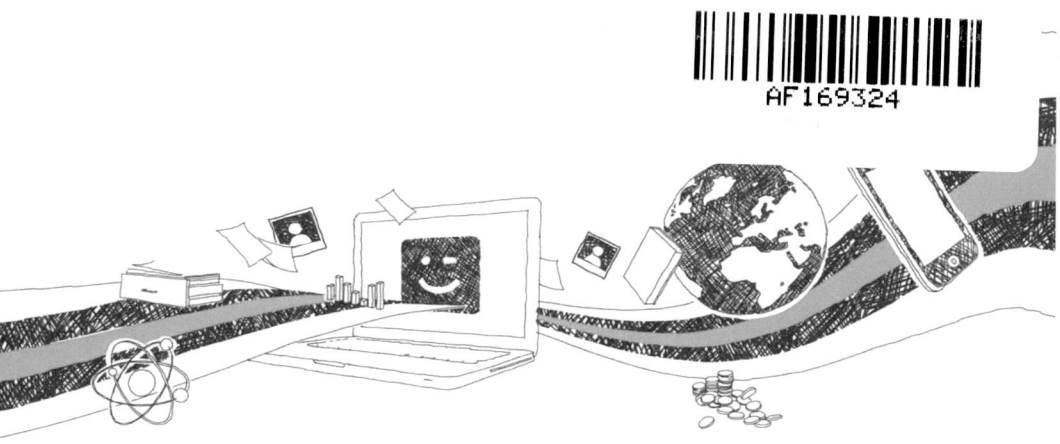

- We will publish your bachelor's and master's thesis, essays and papers

- Your own eBook and book -
  sold worldwide in all relevant shops

- Earn money with each sale

Upload your text at www.GRIN.com
and publish for free

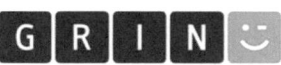

Bibliographic information published by the German National Library:

The German National Library lists this publication in the National Bibliography; detailed bibliographic data are available on the Internet at http://dnb.dnb.de .

This book is copyright material and must not be copied, reproduced, transferred, distributed, leased, licensed or publicly performed or used in any way except as specifically permitted in writing by the publishers, as allowed under the terms and conditions under which it was purchased or as strictly permitted by applicable copyright law. Any unauthorized distribution or use of this text may be a direct infringement of the author s and publisher s rights and those responsible may be liable in law accordingly.

Imprint:

Copyright © 2017 GRIN Verlag, Open Publishing GmbH
Print and binding: Books on Demand GmbH, Norderstedt Germany
ISBN: 9783668576759

This book at GRIN:

http://www.grin.com/en/e-book/381029/ethical-issues-of-human-cloning

Patrick Kimuyu

Ethical Issues of Human Cloning

GRIN Publishing

GRIN - Your knowledge has value

Since its foundation in 1998, GRIN has specialized in publishing academic texts by students, college teachers and other academics as e-book and printed book. The website www.grin.com is an ideal platform for presenting term papers, final papers, scientific essays, dissertations and specialist books.

Visit us on the internet:

http://www.grin.com/

http://www.facebook.com/grincom

http://www.twitter.com/grin_com

ETHICAL ISSUES IN GENETIC ENGINEERING

Name: Patrick K. Kimuyu

Genetic engineering is currently gaining unprecedented popularity owing to its usefulness in solving numerous biological problems. It has become a powerful tool in virtually all biological aspects of life. In medicine, genetic engineering has proven to be reliable in treating and managing biological disorders (Judson, 2001). It has also gained popularity in addressing the challenges posed by chronic diseases such as diabetes. The discovery of the so-called Induced Adult Stem-Cell Therapy and the industrial production of Insulin for treatment of diabetes seem to have shaped the social perspective of genetic engineering. On the other hand, genetic engineering technology has become one of the most reliable biological tools for increasing food production for rapidly growing global population. However, despite the numerous benefits of genetic engineering, immense criticism has emerged, especially with regard to the ethical perspective of the technology. Scientists are in unprecedented dilemma of whether the reproduction of cloned organisms will cause undesirable physical and behavioral traits, leading to the alteration of 'normal' organisms. Currently, there has emerged immense debate on human cloning leading to the shift of ethical perception on genetic engineering. Human cloning is believed to be one of the most popular biotechnological approaches with widespread adoption in the medical field. This is probably so because; it has enabled medical professionals to address some of the most challenging health issues by providing them with extensive medical approach into an array of diseases and health conditions. Some of the medical applications, which have created unprecedented ethical debates among the global population, are the Somatic-cell Nuclear Transfer and test tube baby technology (American Society for Reproductive Medicine, 2012). Therefore, this essay will give an overview on the ethics of human cloning. It will provide a concise summary on the development of cloning and, then discuss the scientific, societal and religious ethical perspectives to the issue.

Concisely, cloning is a biological tool used for medical, industrial production, environmental system control and research. In regard to human cloning, the term Cloning refers to the process of transferring embryonic or adult nuclei from the donor's cell and implanting the genomic code in another cell for the purpose of producing an organism with identical genetic components similar to the donor (McGee, 2001). The new organism with identical genes to the donor is usually referred as the clone. In other words, the clone is a twin organism to the donor since they are identical in virtually all aspects ranging from the genetic composition to behavior and character. Research on cloning is estimated to have begun in early 1950's when some scientists in Pennsylvania achieved a breakthrough in cloning an adult frog from embryonic cell (Logston, n.d). This form of cloning is also known as embryonic twinning and is currently applied in the animal husbandry in the agricultural sector.

Further research studies followed shortly after, but none of them recorded success. In 1980, a group of researchers at the Allegheny University of Health made attempts in cloning a frog from adult red blood cells successfully to produce healthy tadpoles: although the new off-springs died during the metamorphic stages before adult stage. Success in cloning of adult mammals was achieved recently when Scottish scientists cloned the sheep named Dolly. Since then, cloning advanced substantially as a useful tool in medicine and biomedical research (Wilnut et. al 74).

Human cloning has emerged as a controversial ethical issue because of several aspects. One of the most significant aspects, which might have influenced the understanding of scientists over the issue of human cloning, could be its uncertain definition. Currently, cloning in human beings has never been defined precisely. There is no clear distinction between the use of cloning in humans to produce a new off-spring for purposes of procreation or use as a biomedical tool in medicine. In addition, it has been evidenced in the initial research studies that cloning carries fatal implications especially with regard to health risks. McGee (2001) remarks, "Human cloning [is] the most controversial debate of the decade" (1).

In regard to the scientific ethical perspective, cloning has been evidenced to be accompanied with fatal outcomes. The process of genome transfer from the donor individual to the new cell is usually very complex. Therefore, it requires great precautions to avoid inefficient genetic transformation errors. Given the fact that the new off-spring relies solely on the donor as the major source of all genetic components, any inefficiency in the cloning procedure will mean the off-spring is genetically deformed; thus, exposing it to a reduced life expectancy. In case a gene in the donor fails to be efficiently transferred to the new cell; the off-spring will have a deficiency of the missing particular gene. This may be very fatal if the deficient gene plays a major role in the vital body organs such as the brain, liver, heart or the central nervous system.

Moreover, deficiency of genes involved in enzyme biosynthesis, which are involved in metabolic regulatory processes may cause a permanent breakdown of the concerned metabolic process. It has also been noted that contamination of the donor genomic material during the cloning process lead to errors. For instance, the cloning procedures require that the donor DNA material get isolated in the laboratory through an aseptic procedure. If proper procedures are not adopted, this genomic material can be degraded by DNases which are scattered everywhere even on the fingers. As a result, incomplete genomic material can be transferred to the new cell which translates to a great deficiency of the off-springs genetic composition.

Currently, medical professionals are experiencing an unprecedented challenge in correcting the existing genetic disorders. In fact, biomedical research has failed to come up with an effective solution to the majority of genetic disorders such as hemophilia and sickle-cell. Therefore, introduction of some many more genetic related disorders will lead to enormous challenges to our efforts of finding solutions to genetic disorders. Moreover, it might be very dangerous if the off-springs with genetic disorders produced through inefficient cloning procedures are allowed to reproduce freely in nature. This means that artificially generated genetic disorder will circulate in the population and become permanent: usually occurring in individuals along that family tree. A clear example of fatal outcomes of cloning in various organisms can be given by the research done in 1980's by biologists using adult red blood cells of a frog (Logston, n.d). In this experiment, healthy tadpoles were produced but they all died during the subsequent metamorphic processes before reaching the adult stage. This means fatal errors occurred during cloning. It might also mean that, this process is not usually successful in most circumstances. If it were reliable, at least some few tadpoles of the entire population of two hundred and twenty five transformed embryos should have survived to maturity. Unfortunately, they all died, which means; this process is unreliable in human beings at all circumstances.

The second example to prove cloning in mammals inefficient is the Dolly sheep produced in Scotland. Scottish scientists transferred adult udder genomic material from the donor sheep into two hundred and seventy five new cells then incubated to develop into adults. Surprisingly, out of the two hundred and seventy five transformed new cells, dolly sheep was the only survivor. All the other two hundred and seventy four cells failed to develop into adult sheep off-springs (Logston, n.d). More surprisingly, even the survivor; the dolly sheep died some time later, although these scientists claimed that she died of cancer complications. Imagine these were human off-springs! The loss would have been great. Therefore, cloning appears to be accompanied with fatal results, which may put human health at a great risk than the one posed by the current genetic disorders. Despite the critic by some scientists, a large number of biomedical scientists look at it as a useful tool in medicine which holds great promise to saving lives, especially for individuals who are terminally ill. They view this biomedical approach as the only possible way that artificial synthesis of organs, which does not undergo repair after an injury such as the spinal cord can be produced in the laboratory or else in a surrogate individual then transplanted to the donor so as to replace the damaged tissue or organ.

Another significant ethical aspect of human cloning is the unprecedented resistance by the society. From a societal ethical perspective, human cloning is regarded to as a violation of the societal norms and values. Ordinarily, off-springs acquire all their genetic characteristics from their parents. Their sex and other genetic composition are determined by genes in both the father and mother. Therefore, the off-spring is a product of the two individuals. As such, the off-spring is expected to express behavioral characteristics related to those of its father and mother (Dickenson, 2002). Therefore, the identity of the off-spring can be ascertained by analysis of the mother and the father's genome through DNA sequencing. More precisely through the finger-printing genetic procedures, which are based on closeness of the parents' DNA fragments with those of the off-spring (Harris & Holm, 2006). In contrast, in cloning the nuclear donor is usually one, therefore: genetic recombination does not take place in producing the twin off-spring. Another ethical issue related to cloning of human beings lies in the aspect of maintaining the element of sameness in the off-spring (McGee, 2001). Ordinarily, individual are unique in different biological ways. Behavioral characteristics displayed by different individuals vary significantly. The application of human cloning to produce an identical replica brings great uncertainty if all the behavioral characteristics will be displayed in the twin off-spring. Some people would prefer retention of all the outstanding good characteristics such as intelligence, as well as, the good morals that characterize an individual as good. It might be that variations in behavioral characteristics between the donor and the off-spring occur. That will mean, the off-spring is not similar to the donor especially with regard to overall human behavior which encompasses social values and societal norms (Fox, 2001).

However, despite the societal perspective on the issue of human cloning, there is an increasing demand by family members who have their loved ones pinned down by terminal illnesses to have cloning performed to retain a replica of the terminally ill family member. These individuals seem to support human cloning: that is so because they have no other option of curing their friend from complicated illness (Harris & Holm, 2000).

On the other hand, cloning in humans appears unacceptable especially with regard to religious beliefs. It is regarded to as immoral, since; virtually all religions belief that the role of creation is done only by God whom they believe to be the giver of life. In addition, some religions such as Catholics believe in pro-life. As a result, artificial production of human beings is a mortal sin or rather blasphemy because it is seen as competing with God in creation. In general, human cloning violates all the fundamental beliefs of virtually all religions. Surprisingly, majority of biomedical research scientists hold to several religious beliefs. Therefore, they appear to be sinning in a very special manner unknowingly. Despite the observed objection to adoption of human cloning, a large number of both scientists, as well as, members of the public appreciate the invention of cloning technology. Wilnut, a renowned scientist; laud the inventors of cloning and express great hope that, it will bring a significant boost in medicine and biomedical research. Wilnut et.al remark, "We have reached a timely breakthrough in cloning … it will be easier to solve various health challenges we are experiencing today," (261).

In regard to actions to be taken to address ethical issues on human cloning, there are several approaches, which can be reliable to prevent unrealistic criticism and subvert the accrued benefits of the genetic engineering technology. From a personal perspective, genetic engineering, especially with regard to human cloning, there are significant concerns with the future of genetic engineering. It appears that, the technology of human cloning may result into unprecedented bioethical, social and legal issues in the future.

One of the most significant bioethical concerns is the age of the off-spring. It is believed that the human gene undergoes stages of development; thus, its aging corresponds to the aging of an individual. The uncertainty whether the off-spring will manifest the age characteristics of the donor has emerged as an unprecedented dilemma to researchers in the medical field. It is likely that off-springs produced through human cloning may exhibit some age characteristics. This implies that, off-springs, or rather the clones will manifest age characteristics of the donor individual. Therefore, it will be quite surprising to see newborn displaying aging characteristics of its 50 year old donor.

The second bioethical issue, which is related to human cloning technology, is the life expectancy of the off-spring. Ordinarily, cloning encompasses numerous fatalities as it was evidenced with the dolly sheep developed by Scottish scientists. Seemingly, gene incompatibility may result into abnormalities in the off-spring. Biologically, abnormalities are believed to reduce life expectance of an individual. Therefore, abnormalities resulting from human cloning are feared to cause early deaths among the human clones compared to the normal individuals. This appears to influence an individual's quality of life. As a result, this notion may cause unprecedented social harm to cloned individuals, in case this aspect is scientifically proven to be true. Moreover, the clone's social status in the society may be adversely compromised, especially with regard to the real beauty of humanity, which is defined by the differences in physical and behavioral characteristics among human beings.

In regard to the legal issues, human cloning appears to present a substantial challenge to the legal systems of the global community. This is probably so because; legal regulations are designed differently in different countries. Countries design laws related to genetic engineering technology with regard to their requirements and capacity to exploit the technology. For instance, some countries, which experience decline in population growth such as developed countries, are considering the adoption of human cloning as a reliable tool to reverse their demographic trends. As a result, laws related to human cloning seems to enhance the application of the technology. On the other hand, countries, which are experiencing rapid population expansion such as the developing countries, are not supporting the use of human cloning technology, especially with regard to multiplication of individuals from a single donor. This is so because; these countries are experiencing unprecedented social challenges; thus, they are embarking on population control measures. However, most developing countries enact laws, which are aimed at increasing food production. Therefore, there is lack of homogeneity in regulating human cloning technology and, this may lead to a legal conflict among the global community.

In a brief conclusion, human cloning appears to create unprecedented ethical issues among the global population despite its expected benefits in medical applications. There is an immense fear on the future of this technology, especially with regard to the possible undesirable outcomes. However, there are reliable approaches through which the ethical issues related to human cloning can be addressed to reduce their scientific, societal and religious criticism. From a personal perspective, these issues can be solved by a number of recommendations.

First, the uncertainty among scientists over the possible outcomes of human cloning can be lifted by carrying out extensive biomedical research on the biosafety of the technology. This will help to clear doubts on the issue; thus, enabling efficient control of the technology. It is worth noting that, extensive research is the only safe way of preventing the outcome of fatal biological outcomes. In addition, efficient controls of gene activity will ensure that the natural trends in the ecosystem are not influenced by human activities. This can be done in a sterile controlled environment to prevent transmission of genetic materials of the clones into the natural environment.

Secondly, societal ethical issues can be addressed through efficient legal framework, which provides directions on the way human cloning should be conducted. From a sociological perspective, the global population should be give a chance to debate on human cloning so that the laws related to genetic engineering can be designed to suit the interest of the society. Scientists should also educate the public on the benefits of human cloning to clear misconceptions (Nisbet, 2004). In addition, there is a need for the formation of an international agency, which will oversee the application of genetic engineering technologies to ensure homogeneity in legal regulations. As such, countries will enact their laws on genetic engineering with regard to the international standards.

Therefore, human cloning appears to be a useful biotechnological discovery, which holds promise to the eradication of genetic disorders and continuation of genealogies, especially through the use of Somatic-cell Nuclear Transfer. However, stringent measures are required to prevent undesirable outcomes, which may harm the principal tenets of humanity.

Works Cited

American Society for Reproductive Medicine. (2012). Human Somatic Cell Nuclear Transfer and Cloning. *Fertility and Sterility*, *98*(4), 804–7. Retrieved from http://www.asrm.org/uploadedFiles/ASRM_Content/News_and_Publications/Ethics_Committee_Reports_and_Statements/cloning.pdf

Dickenson, D. (2002). *Ethical Issues in Maternal-Fetal Medicine.* Cambridge,UK: Cambridge University Press.

Fox, M. (2001). *Bringing Life to Ethics: Global Bioethics for a Humane Society.* New York, NY: State University of New York Press.

Harris, J., & Holm, S. (2000). The Future of Human Reproduction: Ethics, Choice and Regulation. *J Med Ethics*, *26*, 105-295.

Judson, K. (2001). *Genetic Engineering: Debating the Benefits and Concerns.* Berkeley, NJ: Enslow Pub Incorporated.

Logston, A. (n.d). *The Ethics of Human Cloning.* Retrieved from http://facweb.stvincent.edu/academics/religiousstu/writings/logston1.html

McGee, G. (2001). *Primer on Ethics and Human Cloning.* BioScience Productions, Inc. retrieved from https://people.sunyit.edu/~steve/pos352-w02/class-readings/3.pdf

Nisbet, M. (2004). Public Opinion about Stem Cell Research and Human Cloning. *Public Opin Q.*, *68*(1), 131-154.

YOUR KNOWLEDGE HAS VALUE

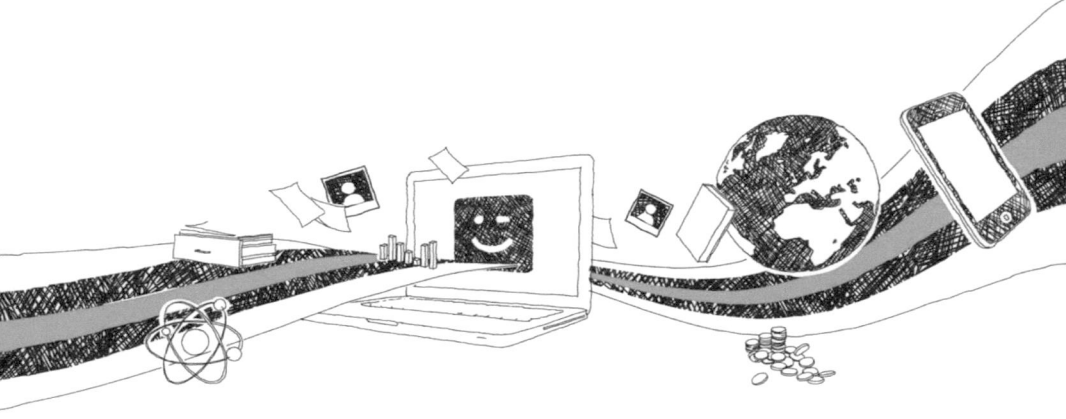

- We will publish your bachelor's and master's thesis, essays and papers

- Your own eBook and book - sold worldwide in all relevant shops

- Earn money with each sale

Upload your text at www.GRIN.com
and publish for free